今日から使える
放射線診療時の英会話

― CD-ROM付 ―

ネイティブスピーカー吹き替えによる
外国人への放射線診療時の対応ムービー

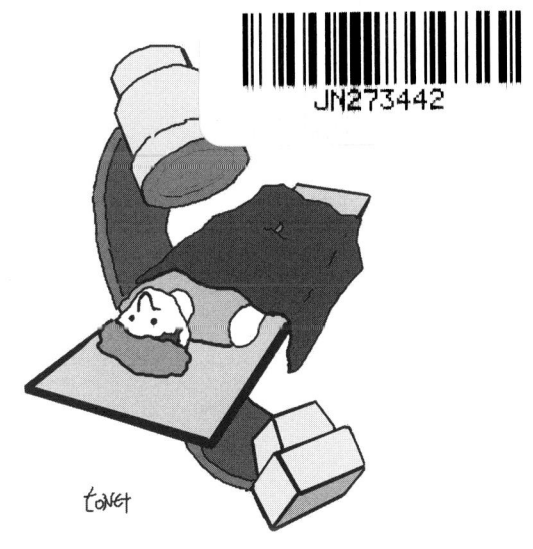

はじめに

　外国人の来院数増加に伴って，診療放射線技師も外国人に接する機会が多くなってきた。すべての放射線技師は，義務教育と高等学校および放射線技師の養成課程で数年間の英語教育を受けており，英語圏の外国人の診療時の対応には事欠かないはずである。しかし，日本での英語教育が，今までは文章を読むことに重点が置かれてきた結果，英作文ができたとしても放射線診療の場合に必要とする英語会話となると自信を持てる人は少ないのではなかろうか。

　アメリカ合衆国南部のフロリダなどでは，移民ができるかぎり早く英語に慣れるように，英語会話の映画に英語会話の字幕スーパーをわざわざ挿入して効果を上げていることを聞いた。このことをヒントに，放射線診療時の映像を撮影し，動きに同期した英語会話の字幕スーパーを配置し，さらに英語圏のネイティブスピーカーに吹き込みを依頼して，外国人に対する放射線診療時の英語会話映像を完成させた。

　数語の会話で自分の意思を患者に伝えたいと考える方もあろうが，簡易な会話は映像中にはできるだけ使用しなかった。しかし，簡単な会話も一度発音を聞いておけば参考になると考え，字幕と音声のみを最後にまとめた。

　また，テキストでは映像中に使用した英語会話を日本語会話と対比するとともに，簡単な会話についてもテキストの後方にまとめて収録した。一度この診療時の英語会話映像を見て練習しておけば，テキストを見るだけで診療時に会話ができるものとの考えから，テキストの大きさは携帯に便利なサイズとした。

この「ネイティブスピーカー吹き替えによる外国人への放射線診療時の対応ムービー」が英語圏患者の対応に役立つことを期待してやまない。なお映像および英語に対しても未熟なため，完璧なものではない。ご意見・ご批判をお寄せいただきたい。

2003年11月

梅崎　典良

　謝辞：この研究に対してご指導，ご協力をいただいた下記の方々にお礼を申し上げます（敬称略）。

英会話講師	Mr. Neil Hall
	Ms. Jennifer Mackay
久留米大学医学部放射線医学教室	石橋　正敏
	馬場　健吉
久留米大学病院画像診断センター	高田　公義
	本野あゆみ
福岡県カナダ領事館	田村　恵美
米国ニューヨークSt. Peter's Hospital	宇佐見良子
久留米大学病院核医学検査室	神代　富江
久留米大学医学部付属医療センター画像センター	金子美奈子
久留米大学医学部フォトセンター	柳　洋一
公立八女総合病院技術部診療放射線	石橋　秀伸
	利根　輝紀
	松雪　公芳
	堤　健治
公立八女総合病院看護部	平井　文代

この作品は、「ネイティブスピーカー吹き替えによる外国人への放射線診療時の対応ビデオ作成研究班」が2001年度の(社)福岡県放射線技師会研究助成金を受けて作成したものです。許可なく、映像、音声などを他に転用することを禁じます。詳細については(社)福岡県放射線技師会までお問い合わせください。

社団法人　福岡県放射線技師会
　〒810‐8505　福岡市中央区赤坂1丁目14番5号
　(財)福岡県看護等研究研修センター内
　　TEL 092‐751‐8428　　FAX 092‐751‐4195
　　e-mail: rt-master@fukuoka-rt.or.jp

Copyright ©2001-2002 the Fukuoka Association of Radiological Technologists. All rights reserved.

This video was created by the Research Group. The production of this correspondence video in radiation medicine which is intended for use by foreigners was dubbed by a native speaker. It was supported by a 2001 Fiscal year research grant courtesy of the Fukuoka Association of Radiological Technologists.

No part of this video may be reproduced including images and audio in any form without permission. Please contact the Fukuoka Association of Radiological Technologists for more details.

e-mail : rt-master@fukuoka-rt.or.jp

研究者

- 久留米大学病院画像診断センター

    中嶋　法忠　　河村　政秀　　前田　孝　　小野　博志

    川田　秀道　　福島　和仁　　谷川　仁　　梨子木一高

    黒木　英郁　　真弓千賀子　　田村　崇　　中村　忍

- 久留米大学病院核医学検査室

    福留　良文　　松藤　次雄　　河村　誠治

- 久留米大学病院放射線治療センター

    執行　一幸

- 久留米大学医学部付属医療センター画像センター

    井口　安則　　宮川　照生　　河村るり子　　神崎　好彦

- 公立八女総合病院技術部診療放射線

    杉山　嘉郎　　宮原　真二　　平田　智徳　　岩村真由美

- 社会保険久留米第一病院

    中原　博子

- 第一薬科大学放射薬品学教室

    梅崎　典良

作品作成者

◎シナリオ・ビデオ撮影

  胸部撮影（_{CD-ROM} 2分44秒）   宮川 照生

  腹部撮影（_{CD-ROM} 2分13秒）   前田 孝

  乳房撮影（_{CD-ROM} 2分54秒）   河村るり子

  胃透視検査（_{CD-ROM} 6分17秒）   平田 智徳

  CT検査（_{CD-ROM} 7分03秒）   河村 政秀

  MR検査（_{CD-ROM} 3分33秒）   川田 秀道

  核医学検査（_{CD-ROM} 3分40秒）   河村 誠治

    骨シンチグラフィ（_{CD-ROM} 1分48秒）

  放射線治療（_{CD-ROM} 2分59秒）   平田 智徳

  放射線の影響（_{CD-ROM} 2分31秒）   執行 一幸

  簡単な会話（_{CD-ROM} 字幕と音声）   小野 博志

◎画像編集   宮原 真二

                   梅崎 典良

◎日英会話テキスト編集   杉山 嘉郎

◎総括   梅崎 典良

                   中嶋 法忠

                   杉山 嘉郎

◎イラスト   利根 輝紀

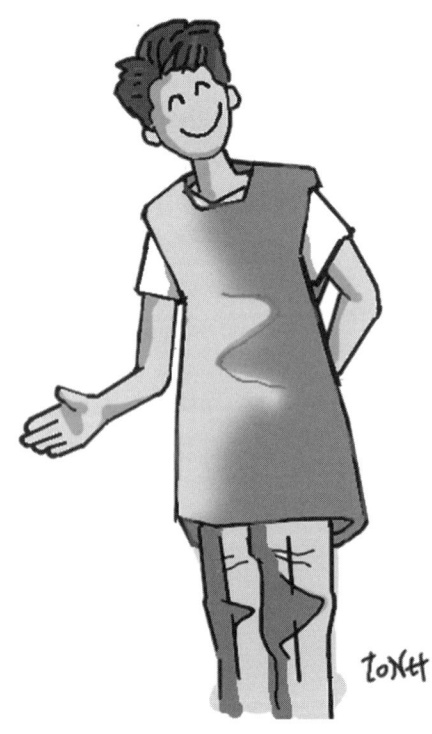

CONTENTS

Chest X-ray　胸部撮影 ·· 11

Abdominal X-ray　腹部撮影 ·· 17

Mammography　乳房撮影 ··· 21

Upper GI Studies　胃透視検査 ······································ 27

CT Examination　CT検査 ··· 37

MR Examination　MR検査 ·· 47

Nuclear Medicine　核医学検査 ······································ 53

　（Bone Scintigraphy　骨シンチグラフィ）

Radiation Therapy　放射線治療 ····································· 63

Influence of Radiation　放射線の影響 ···························· 69

Brief Conversation　簡単な会話 ···································· 75

コラム　湿布とエレキバンの海外事情・16／自己紹介・20／放射線技師の呼称について・26／消化管透視・36／CAT Scan・46／half-lifeについて（1）・52／half-lifeについて（2）・62／英語と米語（1）・68／英語と米語（2）・74

Chest X-ray
胸部撮影

(CD-ROM 2分44秒)

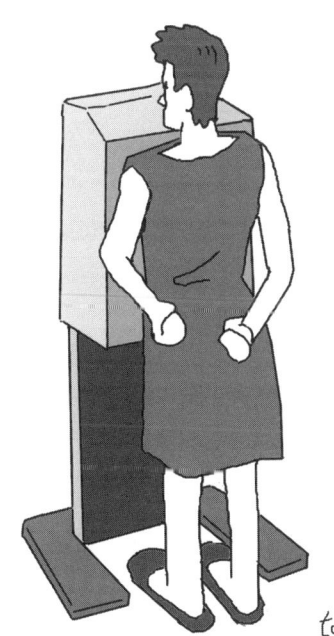

Chest X-ray

Characters

Pt: Patient   Re: Receptionist   RT: Radiological Technologist

Pt Excuse me. Could you tell me where the X-ray reception is please?

Re It's right here.

Would you please give me your hospital I.D. card and the X-ray application form?

So it's a chest X-ray, is that right?

We are going to take the chest X-ray in Room No.1, and they will call you when it's your turn. Please have a seat.

Re Okay, Mr. Smith could you please go to Room No.1.

RT Okay, what I need you to do is take off your clothes and jewellery from the waist up.

We need you to take everything off because if you leave anything on, the X-ray machine will not be able to obtain a precise and accurate X-ray.

Once you have disrobed, please put on this gown and when you are ready, come to the X-ray room.

RT Okay Mr. Smith what I would like you to do is, press your chest firmly against the screen.

Place your hands behind your back.

胸部撮影

登場人物

Pt：患者　Re：受付　RT：放射線技師

Pt　X線検査の受付はどちらですか。

Re　はいこちらです。

撮影申込書と診察カードを一緒に出していただけますか。

胸部撮影ですね。

１番撮影室でお撮りします。順番になりましたらお呼びしますので，１番撮影室の前でしばらくお待ちください。

Re　スミスさん撮影室１番にお入りください。

RT　こちらで，上半身をお脱ぎください。貴金属なども外してください。

それらを身に着けたままでは正確で精度の良いX線写真を撮ることができませんので，ぜひ外してください。

衣服を脱がれたら，このガウンを着て準備ができたらこちらの撮影室に来てください。

RT　こちらの板に胸をつけてください。

両手を腰に持ってきます。

Chest X-ray

RT Push your elbows forward and try to relax your shoulders, and stay still until we say when...

Now take a deep breath and hold your breath 1-2-3-.

Relax and breathe normally.

We need to take one more chest X-ray so...

Please look at me.

Now place your hands behind your head and touch your elbows.

Press your left chest firmly against the screen and stay still until we say when...

Now take a deep breath and hold your breath 1-2-3-.

RT Relax and breathe normally.

Put your clothes back on. Thank you very much.

Everything is finished and you don't need to take anything with you. If you do need some other tests, you will need to go to the reception.

If you don't need any further tests, then please go back to the Main Reception.

Please take all your belongings with you!

Thank you for coming. Take care.

Pt Thank you.

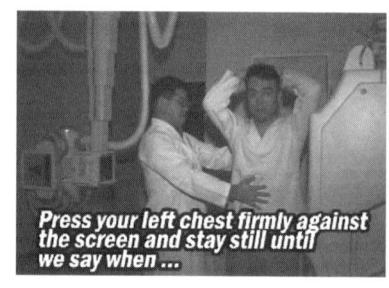
Press your left chest firmly against the screen and stay still until we say when ...

RT 肩の力を抜いて，両肘を突き出します。そのまま，動かないでください。

息を大きく吸い込んでそのまま止めます。

楽にしてください。普通に息をされて結構です。

もう1枚方向を変えて写真を撮ります。

私のほうを見てください。

両手を頭の後ろにもっていきます。それから，両肘をすぼめるようにします。

左胸をできるだけ板にくっつけます。そのまま動かないでください。

息を大きく吸い込んでそのまま止めます。

RT 楽にしてください。普通に息をされて結構です。

衣服を着られても結構です。お疲れさまでした。

検査が終わりました。何も持って行かなくて結構です。もし，他の検査があれば検査受付へ行ってください。

検査がなければ，診療科の受付にお帰りください。

忘れ物がないようにしてください。

お大事に。

Pt ありがとうございました。

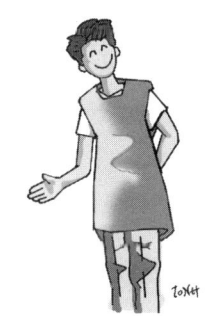

コラム

湿布とエレキバンの海外事情

　このムービーを作成するにあたって「検査前に湿布を取り外す指示はなんと言えばいいの」と協力者である英国人に聞いた。ところが，英国では湿布とかエレキバンはあまり普及していないとのことであった。彼曰く，「湿布とかエレキバンをつけた外人は長年日本に住んでいて，日本語はペラペラだよ」。彼も日本通のようであった。このように外国ではあまり一般的ではない湿布であるが，最近では日本で馴染みの深い湿布を海外でも販売するようになり，TVコマーシャルにも登場しているそうだ。

　では，湿布のことをどのように表現するのだろうか？　一般的な表現方法は"compress"で，冷湿布なら"cold compress"，温湿布なら"hot compress"と言う。ついでに絆創膏は"adhesive plaster"，または"adhesive tape"と言う。

　久光製薬・岡田氏によると，日本で普及している湿布はパップ剤とプラスター剤に大別できるそうだ。パップ剤は白いフェルトの布に水分を含んだ薬を貼付したもので，プラスター剤は薄くて目立たない色で油性の薬剤を使用している。パップ剤の湿布はX線撮影で障害陰影として描出される。プラスター剤は薄いため，さほど障害陰影は発生しない。しかし，原則的には剥がすべきである。ちなみに，パップ剤湿布薬を"gel patch"，プラスター剤湿布薬を単に"patch"と呼んでいるそうだ。

Abdominal X-ray
腹部撮影

(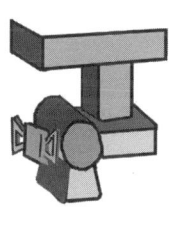 2分13秒)

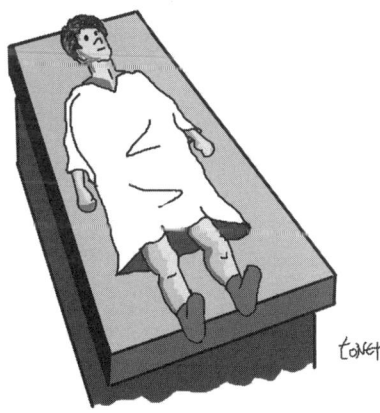

Abdominal X-ray

Characters

RT: Radiological Technologist

RT Miss Yamada, I'm sorry you had to wait so long.
Please come this way.

RT I'm going to take your abdominal X-ray.
Come to this locker room.
Please put on this gown.
Take off any underwear that has buttons or metal.

RT Please step over here.
Take off your shoes and lie on this table on your back.
Please lie straight.
Stay in that position.
Breathe in, breathe out. Hold your breath.

RT Okay, you may breathe.
All right.
Please wait in the corridor until we check the film.
Take care, Miss Yamada.

腹部撮影

登場人物

RT：放射線技師

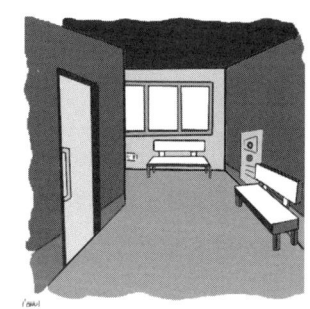

RT　山田さん，お待たせしました。
　　こちらへ来てください。

RT　今から腹部の撮影をします。
　　こちらの更衣室へどうぞ。
　　この服に着替えてください。
　　金具やボタンのついている下着は脱いでください。

RT　こちらへ来てください。
　　靴を脱いで，このテーブルの上に仰向きに横になってください。
　　身体をまっすぐにします。
　　そのまま動かないでください。
　　息を吸って，吐き出して，そのまま止めてください。

RT　息をして楽にしてください。
　　終わりました。
　　写真を確認しますので，しばらく廊下でお待ちください。
　　お大事に，山田さん。

コラム

自己紹介

　このところ，どの病院でも職員は胸に名札をつけている。昭和30年ごろには，この名札着用の習慣はなかった。

　あるとき，放射線技師全員（当時はX線技師）に名札をつけるようにとの達しがあった。あちこち，うろうろして名前を覚えられることに抵抗を感じたが，名札をつけることで，ちょっと有名人になったような気がしたものだ。それまで名札着用の習慣がなかったのがおかしいのかもしれない。名札をつけていることで確かにいろんな人の顔と名前が覚えやすくなった。

　名札着用の効果は，好感が持てる，責任を持つことにあるらしい。外国では，患者さんと対応するとき，放射線技師も自己紹介をする習慣があるようだ。日本でも，主治医，看護師は以前から受け持ち患者に自己紹介していた。自己紹介は，患者との信頼関係をつくる。最近では，放射線治療，核医学，CT，MRI担当の放射線技師も患者さんに自己紹介する習慣が生まれつつある。自己紹介はインフォームド・コンセントへの第一歩なのだ。これからは，一般撮影でも患者さんの名前を呼んで，自己紹介することになるだろう。

(Rt)　Mr. Tanaka. Hello. How are you?
(Pt)　Fine. Thank you, and you?
(Rt)　I'm fine too. Thank you.
　　　My name is Satoh 〜 . I'm a Radiological Technologist.

Mammography
乳房撮影

(🔊 2分54秒)

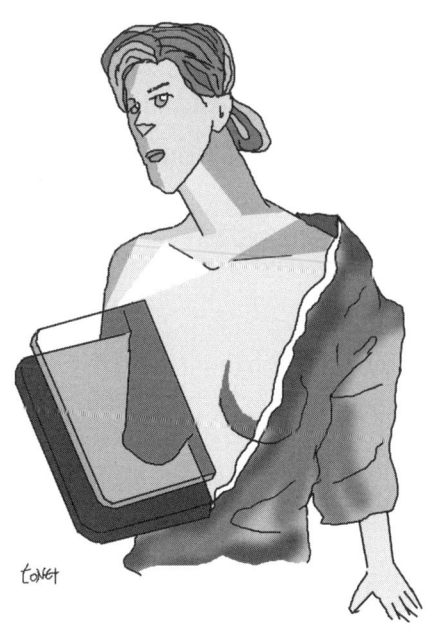

Mammography

Characters

Pt: Patient   RT: Radiological Technologist

RT Mrs. Smith, please come in to the mammography room. Have you ever done a mammography before?

Pt No, I haven't had one before.
Should I take my top clothes off?

RT Yes please. After you have taken off your clothes, wrap this bath towel around your body and please wait.

RT By the way, what reason did you come to the hospital today?

Pt I found a tumor on my breast but it doesn't hurt.

RT Now, we're going to take your mammography from the front and an oblique picture too. Also press your breast to be clear, and could you let me know now if you feel any pain.
Please put your right breast on this board right in the middle and put it inside as much as possible.
Could you hold your face to the left and put your left arm in front and hold the machine please?
I'm going to press your breast.
Are you still okay?

Pt I'm fine.

乳房撮影

登場人物

Pt：患者　RT：放射線技師

RT　スミスさん乳房撮影室へお入りください。
　　乳房撮影は初めてですか？

Pt　はい，初めてです。
　　上半身裸になりますか？

RT　はい。脱がれたらバスタオルを掛けてお待ちください。

RT　その前に，今日はどんな理由で受診しましたか？

Pt　乳房にしこりを見つけました。痛みはありません。

RT　では，今から乳房の撮影をします。正面と斜めの撮影をしますが，お乳のなかが良く見えるように圧迫しますので，痛かったら教えてください。

　　右のお乳をこの台の真んなかに乗せてください。できるだけ乳房の内側を入れるようにして乗せてください。
　　顔は左を向いて，左手は伸ばして機械の取っ手を持ってください。

　　圧迫します。
　　まだ我慢できますか？

Pt　大丈夫です。

Mammography

RT Now, I'm going to take your mammography, so please hold your breath.

Please relax.

Next, I'm going to take from an oblique angle.

Could you move your left breast outside by your left hand.

RT I'm going to take your mammography, so please hold your breath.

Please relax.

Everything is done.

I'm going to develop these films and check them.

Could you wait a moment please?

You can put your clothes back on.

Pt Where should I go next?

RT If these films are fine, you can go back to the Main Reception, and please take care.

乳房撮影

RT では，撮影しますので，息を止めてください。

楽にしてください。
次は，斜めから撮影します。
左手で左胸を外側に押してください。

RT では，撮影します。息を止めてください。

楽にしてください。
終わりました。
フィルムを現像し，写真の写り具合をチェックします。
しばらく待っていただけませんか。
衣服を着ても良いですよ。

Pt 次に，私はどこへ行けばいいんですか。
RT 写真がよく写っていたら，受診科の受付にお帰りください。お大事に。

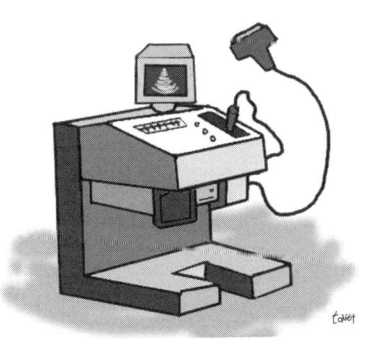

コラム

放射線技師の呼称について

　日本の放射線技師会は，放射線技師の英語表記について"Radiological Technologist"としているが，外国ではどのような呼ばれ方をしているのだろうか。インターネットで検索してみた。

　アメリカ　　Radiologic Technologist, Radiographer
　イギリス　　Radiographer
　カ ナ ダ　　Radiological Technologist, Radiation Therapist, Nuclear MedicineTechnologist, Magnetic Resonance Technologist
　オーストラリア　Radiographer, Radiation Therapist
　ニュージーランド　Medical Radiation Technologist, Radiation Therapist
　シンガポール　Radiographer
　マ レ ー シ ア　Radiographer
　香　　港　Radiographer
　タ　　イ　Radiological Technologist
　台　　湾　Radiologic Technologist

　身分や資格制度がよくわからないため，どこまで正確に示しているか疑問である。特にアメリカの状況は複雑で，さまざまな教育プログラムや専門教育制度が存在し，理解するのは容易ではない。"Radiologic Technologist"と"Radiographer"の違いは診療放射線技師と診療X線技師の違いに近いものだと思われるが，そのほか，"Radiologic Technologist"からの専門資格として"Cardiovascular-Interventional Technologist"，"Computed Tomography Technologist"，"Magnetic Resonance Technologist"，"Nuclear Medicine Technologist"などがあり，本当にわからない。ただし，放射線技師の呼称としては，一般的には"Radiological Tecnologist"で通用するようだ。

Upper GI Studies
胃透視検査

(💿 6分17秒)

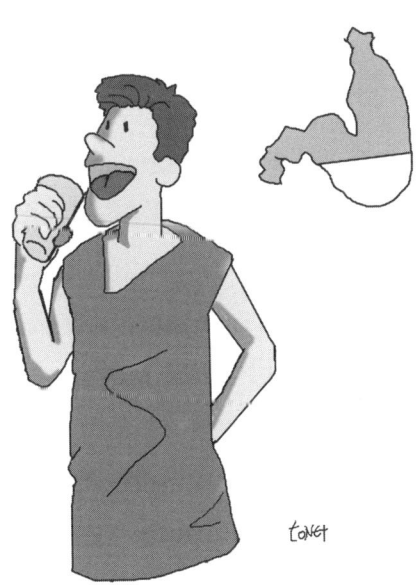

Upper GI Studies

Characters

Pt: Patient   Re: Receptionist   Ns: Nurse   RT: Radiological Technologist

Pt Do you do upper GI's here?
Re Yes, may I have your name?
Pt My name is Mr. Hirata.
Re I see, it's reserved.
Please wait in front of the fluoroscopy room until a nurse calls your name.

◇   ◇

Ns Mr. Hirata, please come in.
May I have your Name and Date of Birth for confirmation?
Pt Off course. My name is Hirata and the date of birth is May 5th 1970.
Ns Okay, please change into these clothes.
You don't need to take off your underwear. But, if you are wearing things made of metal, please take them off.
Please sit down here.
Then, I will give you an intramuscular injection to slow the movement of your stomach.
Before I do so, have you ever suffered from any illness such as high blood pressure, glaucoma, prostate gland enlargement?

胃透視検査

登場人物

Pt：患者　Re：受付　Ns：看護師　RT：放射線技師

Pt　胃透視検査はこちらですか？

Re　はい。あなたのお名前はなんとおっしゃるのですか。

Pt　平田と言います。

Re　わかりました。予約されていますね。
　　それでは，看護師がお呼びするまで，そちらの透視室の前でお待ちください。

Ns　平田さん，なかにお入りください。
　　確認のため，お名前と生年月日を教えてもらって良いですか。

Pt　はい。名前は平田で，生年月日は1970年5月5日です。

Ns　それではこちらで服を脱いでこの服に着替えてください。
　　下着は着ていても良いですよ。もし金属やプラスチック類がついていたら脱いでください。
　　こちらにお座りください。
　　今から胃の動きを止める注射をします。

　　今までに高血圧，緑内障，前立腺肥大などと言われたことはないですか？

Upper GI Studies

Pt No, I've never had any of those.

Ns Then, I'll inject it into your shoulder.

Please wait a little while until the medicine becomes effective.

◇   ◇

RT Mr. Hirata, please stand on this board.

I'm going to start the stomach fluoroscopy now.

At first, hold this barium container with your left hand.

Please turn in a left diagonal direction.

Please hold a mouthful of this liquid in your mouth, and swallow it when I give you a signal.

Okay, please swallow it.

Then please turn to the front and drink the remainder.

Okay, please swallow it.

Did you drink it all?

Pt Yes.

RT I would like you to take this medicine for inflating your stomach. Please put this granule in your mouth first, and swallow the granule with this water. I think that you will probably feel like burping, but please endure it until this test is finished.

RT The table becomes level.

Please spin around to the right three times quickly.

Please turn in a left diagonal direction.

胃透視検査

Pt　ありません。

Ns　それじゃ，肩に注射をします。
　　それではここに腰かけて少し待っててください。

RT　平田さん，この台にお上がりください。
　　それでは今から検査を始めます。
　　まず左手でそのコップを持って，左斜めを向いてください。

　　一口多めに口に含んで，合図をしたら飲んでください。

　　はい，飲み込んでください。
　　それでは正面を向いて残りを飲んでください。
　　はい，飲み込んでください。
　　すべて飲み込みましたか。

Pt　はい。

RT　胃を膨張させるためにこの薬を飲んでください。最初にこの粉を口にためて，この水で一気に流し込んでください。げっぷが出やすくなりますけど検査が終わるまでげっぷを我慢してください。

RT　ベッドを倒します。
　　それでは右回りですばやく3回まわってください。
　　左斜め向きになります。

Upper GI Studies

RT Breathe out and hold your breath for a second.

Relax please.

Please spin around to the right once again.

Please turn to the left a little, and breathe out a little and hold.

Relax please.

Please hold on to the handrail with both hands and turn to the right a little.

Please breathe in, and inflate your stomach and hold.

Relax please.

Please turn to the right side, and stay still.

Please grasp the handrails with both hands and touch your right waist, and keep a posture of oblique.

Breathe in and inflate your stomach and hold.

Relax please.

Please turn over on your back from the left, and turn to the right oblique.

Breathe in and hold.

Relax please.

Please turn to the right side and hold up both your hands.

Breathe in and hold.

Relax please.

Please turn to the front.

Now I will press your abdomen. If you feel a pain, please let me know.

胃透視検査

RT　息を吐いて，そこで息を止めます。
　　楽にしてください。
　　もう一度右回りで1回転してください。
　　少し左を向いて，そこで軽く息を吐いて止めます。

　　楽にしてください。
　　横の手すりを持って，少し右斜め向きになります。

　　そこで息を吸ってお腹を大きく膨らませ，息を止めます。
　　楽にしてください。
　　右側からうつ伏せになります。
　　横の手すりを持って，右側を浮かせて斜め向きになります。

　　息を大きくすってお腹を膨らませ，そこで息を止めます。
　　楽にしてください。
　　左側から仰向けになってください。次に右斜め向きになります。

　　息を吸って，止めます。
　　楽にしてください。
　　今度は左の真横向きになって両手をあげます。
　　息を吸って，止めます。
　　楽にしてください。
　　正面向きになります。
　　今からお腹を押さえますので，もし痛かったら言ってください。

Upper GI Studies

RT Do you feel any pain?
Pt No I don't.
RT Hold your breath.
   Now it is finished.
   Please drink a lot of water today, because this will help in emptying your bowels as soon as possible.

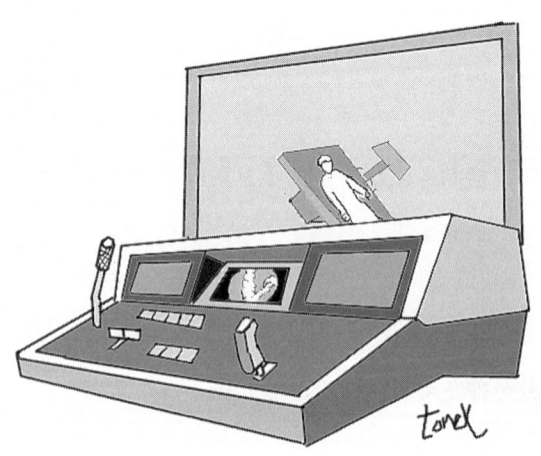

胃透視検査

RT 痛くないですか。

Pt 大丈夫です。

RT そこで息を止めます。

お疲れさまでした。

今日は水分を多めにとって，早めに便を出すようにしてください。

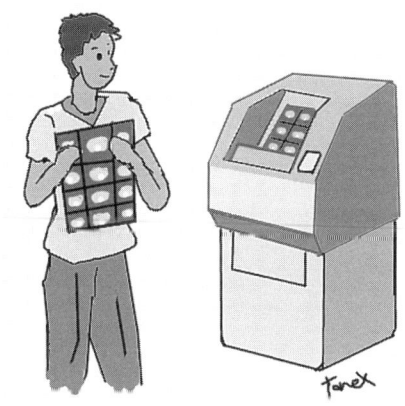

コラム

消化管透視

　上部消化管透視は英語で"Upper Gastrointestinal Studies"または"Upper Gastrointestinal Series"と言い，略して"UGI's"である。検査の前処置を説明する場合は，

　Nothing to eat, drink, or chew, and no smoking, after 11 P.M. the night before appointment.

といった表現が例としてあげられる。

　バリウム造影剤は"contrast material called barium"，発泡剤は"baking-soda crystals"といった表現もできる。二重造影検査は"air-contrast"または"double-contrast"である。

　ちなみに，下部消化管透視は"Lower Gastrointestinal Studies"または"Lower Gastrointestinal Series"となり，小腸から大腸までの検査を示す。ただし，注腸検査は"Barium Enema"と言うことが多い。

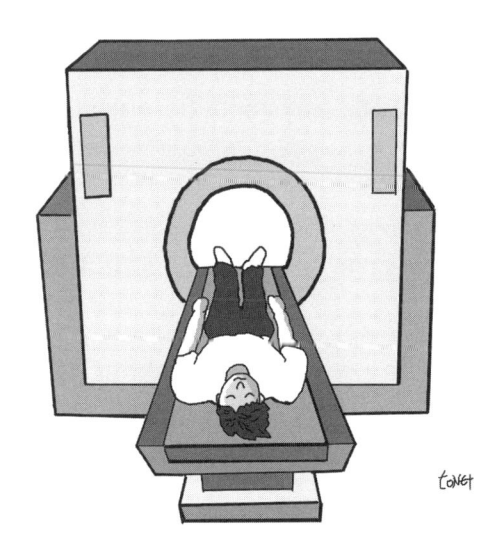

CT Examination
CT検査

(🖸 7分03秒)

CT Examination

Characters

Pt: Patient   Re: Receptionist   RT: Radiological Technologist

Pt Is this the place I can have a CT examination?

Re Are you Mr. Nakamura?

Please wait in the reception room that is located on your right hand side.

Pt How long do I have to wait?

Re About ten minutes.

◇   ◇

RT Mr. Nakamura please come in to this examination room.

Now you are going to have an abdominal CT examination.

Please change in to this examination robe.

If you are wearing any metallic objects, please take them off.

RT I'm going to give you some instructions about this CT examination.

The examination will only take about twenty minutes.

You will be given a contrast media injection during this examination.

I will explain about the contrast media injection.

This contrast media injection has some side effects.

CT検査

登場人物

Pt：患者　Re：受付　RT：放射線技師

Pt　CT検査はこちらでしょうか？
Re　中村さんですね。
　　右に進んで，待合室でお待ちください。

Pt　どれくらい待たなければならないのでしょうか。
Re　10分ぐらいです。

　　　　　　　　◇　　　　◇

RT　中村さん，どうぞこの検査室にお入りください。
　　今から，あなたのお腹のCT検査を始めます。

　　この，検査着に着替えてください。
　　もし金属類のついた衣類があれば，お脱ぎください。

RT　今から，検査の説明をいたします。

　　検査はおよそ20分で終わる予定です。
　　今回は，造影剤を注射する検査になっております。

　　造影剤について説明します。
　　この薬は副作用の少ない薬です。

CT Examination

RT I have a report from your doctor that you don't have any particular problems with this contrast media injection. However, if you feel anything unusual during this examination, please tell us so immediately with a loud voice. With this contrast media injection, some people may feel nausea, breathlessness, respiratory problems and itching. Also some people may feel a slight warming sensation. These are some of the small side effects that can be caused by the contrast media injection. But you don't need to worry about this.

During the scanning, I will ask you to hold your breath. I will ask you to breathe in, and then hold your breath for about ten seconds.

You will hear some instructions from the speakers in the room. Please hold your breath properly, until you are told to relax.

Until the CT examination is completed, please stay still as much as you can.

If you cannot hold the posture anymore, please tell us so before you move.

Are there any questions?

Pt I cannot hold my breath for a long time.

RT That's okay, we'll manage.

CT検査

RT　あなたの主治医から造影剤を注射することに問題ないと聞いています。
　　しかし，万一気分が悪くなったら，大きな声でお知らせください。

　　症状は，吐き気，息苦しさ，呼吸異常，かゆみなどがあります。

　　また，この薬により，身体が熱く感じます。
　　しかし，これは造影剤による些細な副作用で，心配することはありません。

　　撮影時には，息を止めていただきます。
　　大きく息を吸って，およそ10秒ぐらい止めてください。

　　合図は，スピーカーから聞こえます。楽にしてくださいと案内するまでは，しっかり止めていてください。

　　予定の検査が終了するまで，身体をできるだけ動かさないでください。
　　もし，我慢できない場合は，動く前にお知らせください。

　　よろしいですか？
Pt　私は息を長く止められません。
RT　はい，わかりました。

CT Examination

RT Please lay down on this bed.
   Please put your head on this pillow.
   Please put your legs on here, and lay on your back.
   Please raise your hands and leave them by the side of your head. You will have a CT examination in this posture.
   Are you comfortable in this position?
   Now I'm going to raise the bed position.
   Then put you in the starting position.
   Now we will begin the CT examination.

RT Please follow the instructions to control your breathing.
   Now let's start.
   Please breathe in, and then hold your breath.
   Now you can breathe out.
   Are you all right?
   Now we are going to inject the back of your hand with the contrast media injection.
   Please follow the Doctor's instructions.

RT Let's start the injection.
   Breathe in, and then hold your breath.
   Relax please.

RT Now your CT examination is over.

CT検査

RT　それではこのベッドに寝てください。
　　頭はこの枕に乗せてください。
　　足をこの上に乗せて，仰向けに横になってください。
　　両手をあげて頭の横に置いてください。この状態で検査をします。

　　大丈夫ですか？
　　それではベッドが上がります。
　　位置を合わせます。
　　それでは撮影を始めます。

RT　息止めの合図に従ってください。
　　それでは始めます。
　　息を吸って止めてください。
　　楽にしてください。
　　大丈夫ですか？
　　それでは次に，手に造影剤を注射します。

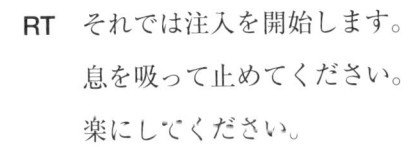

　　医師の指示に従ってください。

RT　それでは注入を開始します。
　　息を吸って止めてください。
　　楽にしてください。

RT　すべての検査は終了しました。

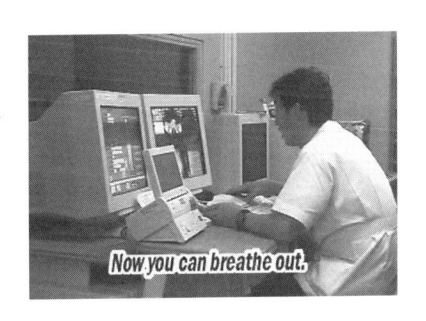

CT Examination

RT Are you all right?

Now I'll lower the bed position for you.

You can sit up now.

Your Doctor is going to tell you the results of this CT examination.

RT Because you had a contrast media injection, please drink water a bit more than usual.

If you have anything unusual such as rush within a couple of days, please consult the hospital.

It might be an side effect of the contrast media injection you had today.

If you have any questions, do not hesitate to ask your Doctor.

Now you can change your clothes.

See you Mr. Nakamura, and take care of yourself.

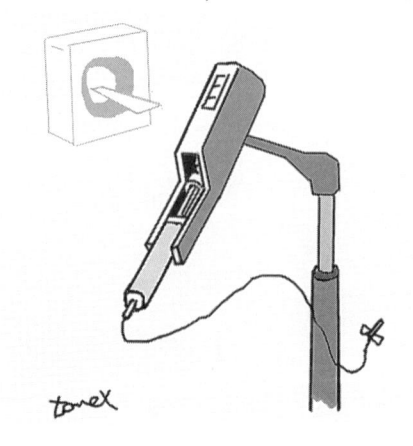

RT 大丈夫ですか？
ベッドを安全な位置に戻します。
それでは，起きてください。
検査結果は，主治医が説明します。

RT 今日は造影剤を使用しておりますので，水分を多くおとりください。
今後，数日のうちに，発疹や身体の変調があった場合は病院に連絡してください。
造影剤の影響も考えられます。

詳しくは，受診科でお尋ねください。

着替えをしてください。
お大事に。

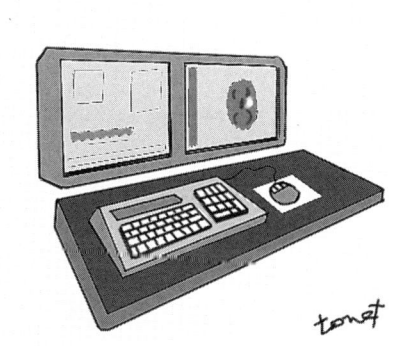

コラム

CAT Scan

　このムービー作成にあたって，協力者の英国人から「向こうではCTのことをCAT Scanとも言うが，これは何の略なのか」と逆に質問された。米英では一般的に使われているようで，米国の医療サイトを調べていても，CT検査の説明で次のような言葉によく出会う。

　Computed tomography—sometimes called CAT scan—

　"Computer Aided Tomography"の略かなとも思ったが，よく調べてみると"Computed Axial Tomography"の略であることがわかった。略する前の言葉を比べると"Computed Axial Tomography"のほうが直感的にわかりやすいと思われるし，略号にしても発音しやすいと思うのは私だけだろうか？

　ところで，CT検査の説明はどのように表現されているのだろうか。ACR RSNAのホームページには次のような解説が載せられている。

Uses special x-ray equipment to obtain image data from different angles around the body, then uses computer processing of the information to show a cross-section of body tissues and organs.

MR Examination
MR検査

(💿 3分33秒)

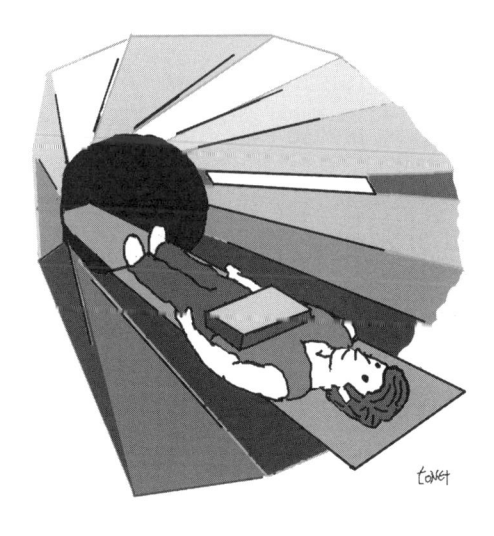

MR Examination

Characters

Pt: Patient   RT: Radiological Technologist

RT Hello! Are you Miss Chikako Mayumi?
Excuse me for asking, but how much do you weigh?
Today we are going to examine your brain.
Please wait in the waiting room over there, while we prepare for the examination.

RT Have you ever had a heart or brain operation?
Please take off any metals, such as hairpins, necklaces, earrings and watches.
If you have any valuables, like a wallet, purse or watch can you put them in a locker please.
If you are wearing underwear with any kind of metal including wires, please take them off too. You can change into this robe.
When you are ready, please lock the locker, sit in this chair and wait.

◇   ◇

RT Thank you for waiting, Miss Mayumi.
Please come in from this way.
You can put the locker key here.
The machine makes a lot of noise, so please wear these earplugs.

MR検査

登場人物

Pt：患者　RT：放射線技師

RT　真弓ちかこさんですか。
　　失礼ですが体重を教えてください。
　　本日は脳の検査をする予定です。
　　準備がありますので，そちらの待合い室でお待ちください。

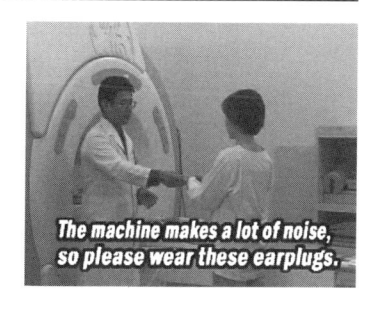

RT　心臓や脳の手術を受けたことがありますか。
　　ヘアピン，ネックレス，ピアス，時計など，金属を身に着けておりましたら外しておいてください。
　　財布，腕時計などの貴重品もロッカーに入れておいてください。

　　また，下着にも金属などがついていましたら，こちらの検査衣にお着替えください。

　　用意ができましたら，ロッカーの鍵をかけて，こちらの椅子に腰かけてお待ちください。

　　　　　　◇　　　◇

RT　真弓さん，お待たせいたしました。
　　どうぞこちらからお入りください。
　　ロッカーの鍵はこちらへ置いてください。
　　機械の音が大きいので，耳栓をしてください。

MR Examination

RT Please lie down here. Your head this way. Your feet the other way.
　　The examination lasts for about twenty minutes.
　　Please do not move during the examination.
　　If you start to feel sick or queasy, please let us know using a loud voice or by holding this ball tightly.
　　Are you okay?

RT The laser light is coming out, so please keep your eyes closed. Now we are starting the examination.
　　Miss Mayumi, we are starting the examination and there will be a loud noise. Please don't move and listen to me.

RT Right now, you will be given an injection with a medicine that makes lesions.
　　About ten minutes after the injection, the examination will be finished.
　　The examination is finished now.

RT I will bring out a table, so please wait there and keep still.
　　Miss Mayumi, are you okay?
　　Are you feeling fine?
　　If you don't have any other examinations after this, please go back to the clinical department that there.
　　Take care.

MR検査

RT　頭をこちらにして，ベッドに横になってください。

　　検査時間はおよそ20分ぐらいです。
　　検査中は体を動かさないでください。
　　もし，検査途中で気分が悪くなったりしたら大声を出すか，このボールを強く握ってください。
　　よろしいですか。

RT　レーザー光が出ていますので目を閉じていてください。それでは検査を始めます。
　　真弓さん，検査を始めます。大きな音がします。体を動かさないようにして聞いてください。

RT　今から，検査目的部位がよく写るお薬を注射します。

　　注射が終わりましたら10分ぐらいで検査を終わります。

　　検査終わりました。

RT　テーブルを出しますのでそのままお待ちください。
　　真弓さん，大丈夫ですか。
　　気分は悪くないですか。
　　この後，他に検査がなければおかかりの診療科でお待ちください。

　　お大事にしてください。

コ ラ ム

half-life について（1）

　半減期（half-life）という言葉は，われわれの業界では耳慣れた言葉で当然のように使用している。しかし，患者さんに説明するとき，半減期という部分になると怪訝な顔をされる。調査してわかったことであるが，どのように書くのか，また何を言っているのかわからないとのことであった。これは，外国人にもあてはまりそうである。

　英英辞書によるとhalf-lifeは，

　　　time after which radioactivity etc. is half its original value.

と書いてあった。また，教科書では，次のような説明がある。

　　　The decay rate could be expressed in terms of a half-life, which is the time it takes for the radioactivity of a radioelement to decay to one-half of its original value.

　インターネットで調べていると，

　　　What's half-life mean you ask?

という文章が見つかった。外国人も困っているらしい。答を紹介する。

　　　half-life: The time required for half a sample of radioactive nuclei to decay.

　また，薬学分野では「生体内の薬物濃度が，代謝・排泄されて半分になるのに要する時間」と記されていた。

　雑誌にも半減期という言葉がある。意味は，よく理解できないが，現在からさかのぼって全引用文献数の累計値が50％になる年を雑誌の半減期（half-life）と言うらしい。引用している文献の半減期を引用半減期（citing half-life），引用されている文献の半減期（cited half-life）というように使用する。

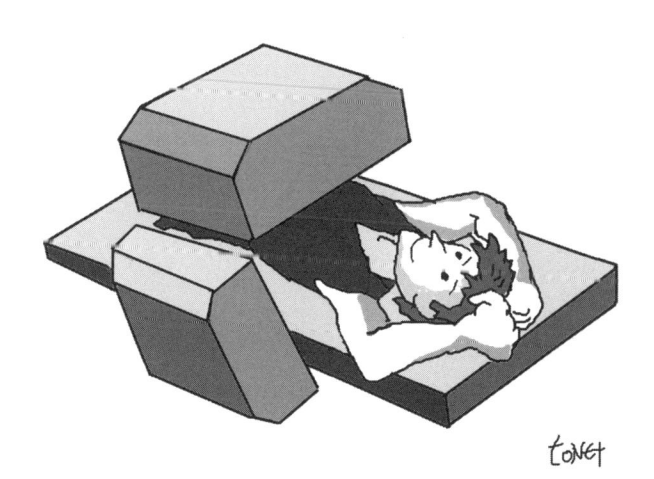

Nuclear Medicine
核医学検査

(CD-ROM 3分40秒)

Bone scintigraphy　骨シンチグラフィ

(CD-ROM 1分48秒)

Nuclear Medicine

Characters

Patient   Receptionist   Radiological Technologist   Doctor

Pt Excuse me, is this the reception window of the Radiological Room?

Re Yes it is, may I have your name please?

Pt My name is Mr. Smith.

Re Mr. Smith, you are supposed to receive a bone scintigraphy.

Mr. Smith, if you could please take off your shoes and put on a pair of yellow slippers. Then, enter the examination room and give your name to the technician in charge at the treatment chamber. There you will also receive an injection with radioactive medicine.

◇   ◇

RT Excuse me, may I have your name please?

Pt Yes, my name is Mr. Smith.

RT What we are going to do today, is give you an injection with radioactive medicine. So could you please put on a pair of yellow slippers and then enter the treatment chamber.

核医学検査

登場人物

Pt：患者　Re：受付　RT：放射線技師　Dr：医師

Pt　核医学検査室の受付はこちらでしょうか。

Re　はいそうです。お名前を教えてください。
Pt　スミスです。
Re　スミスさんは骨シンチグラフィを行うようになっています。

　　ここで下履きから黄色のスリッパに履き替えて検査室へ入っていただき，処置室で担当の技師にお名前をおっしゃってください。そこで検査のための放射性医薬品を注射します。

◇　　　◇

RT　申し訳ありませんがお名前を教えてください。
Pt　スミスです。
RT　ここで検査のための放射性医薬品を注射しますので黄色のスリッパに履き替えて，検査室にお入りください。

Nuclear Medicine

Dr Okay, so we are going to give you an intravenous injection now because you're having a bone scintigraphy today. Please give me your arm. Once you have had your injection, we will need to give you a quick check up three to four hours after the injection. Now it's nine o'clock (9 a.m.), so we will examine you again around one o'clock (1 p.m.). Don't worry about the brief examination it isn't painful at all, and all you have to do is lie down on the bed for about fifteen minutes.

Pt Is there anything important I need to know about, before one o'clock.

RT Well, if you don't have anymore tests after this one, then please eat a normal lunch. Also try to drink as much water as possible because this will aid the quality of the examination results. We will return here at one o'clock for the brief examination.

RT Mr. Smith, how are you feeling? Good! What we need for your test, is for you to go to the toilet please. We've found that if a patient empty's his bladder before the tests, it increase the tests accuracy.

RT Mr. Smith, if you could please lie down on the bed with your head facing here please.

核医学検査

Dr 今日は骨シンチグラフィグラフィを行いますので，静脈注射をいたします。すいませんが，肘を出してください。注射後3～4時間で検査を行います。今は午前9時ですから午後1時から検査を行います。検査はベッドで約15分間横になって行う楽な検査です。

Pt 午後1時まで何か気をつけることはありますか。

RT この検査のみで他の検査がないときは，昼食をおとりください。また，普通より多めに水分摂取をしていただくことで検査の質を高めることができます。それでは，午後1時から検査しますのでよろしくお願いいたします。

RT スミスさん，今から行う検査は膀胱に尿がたまっていないほうが良い検査ができますので，トイレで排尿していただけませんでしょうか。

RT スミスさん，この検査寝台の左を頭にして仰向けに横になってください。

Nuclear Medicine

RT Now, we are going to strap you loosely to the bed, to make sure you don't fall off. Then the gamma camera will come towards you, please don't worry. If the camera touches you, it will automatically stop.

Pt The tests were easier and quicker than I expected. Thank you very much.

RT Okay, Mr. Smith, if you could please go and sit down on the bench, and we'll bring the tests results over to you as quickly as possible.

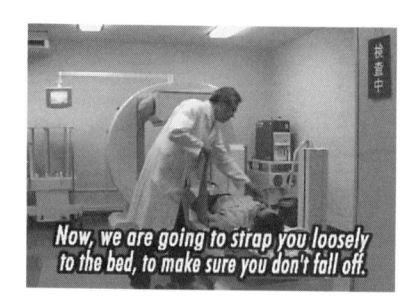

核医学検査

RT　申し訳ありませんが，検査台から落ちないように軽くバンドで固定しておきます。ガンマカメラが体に接近しますが良い検査をするためです。また，万一体にガンマカメラが接触した場合はガンマカメラは自動的に静止します。

Pt　思っていたより楽な検査で早く終わりましたね。ありがとうございました。

RT　検査結果をお渡ししますので，しばらくお待ちください。

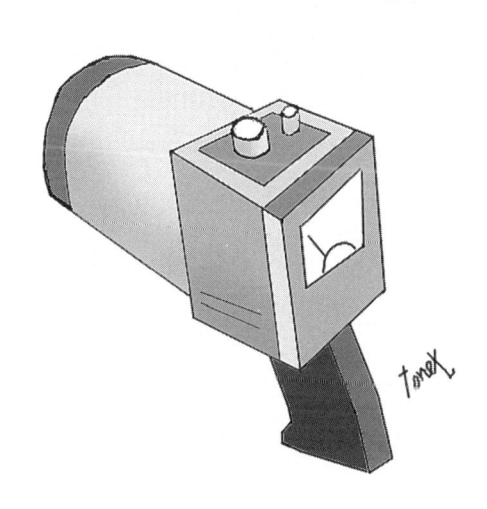

Nuclear Medicine

[About Bone Scintigraphy]

Dr Hello! I'm Doctor Ishibashi, I'm with the Department of Radiology, School of Medicine, at Kurume University.
Bone scintigraphy is a nuclear medical test most frequently used for the diagnosis of bone metastasis.
In this country, bone scintigraphy is now given to more than five hundred thousand patients a year.
This test has a great advantage of being able to examine the whole body without causing any pain and only by administrating a radiopharmaceutical.
But the test has a disadvantage because the costs are very high compared with other image tests, like the chest X-ray, CT and MRI examinations.
However, the sensitivity of the bone scintigraphy to detect bone metastasis is very high so that the test is superior, especially in diagnosing at an early stage.
In addition, the radiopharmaceutical's life span (half-life) is as short as six hours since Tc-99m is used as the radionuclide and radiation exposure is thus very low.
Bone scintigraphy is a safe and non-painful test. So please don't worry about the test.

核医学検査

［**骨シンチグラフィ**について］

Dr　久留米大学医学部・放射線医学講座，石橋と申します。

骨シンチグラフィは，がんの骨転移診断が主な目的となっており，核医学検査のなかで最も多く行われている検査です。
わが国では年間50万件以上の検査が行われています。

また骨シンチグラフィの最大の利点は，放射性医薬品を投与するのみで患者さんに苦痛を与えることなく全身検査が可能なことです。
欠点は，胸部X線写真，CT，MR検査と比較して検査費用が高額なことであると思います。

しかし，骨シンチグラフィにおける骨転移診断の感度は非常に高く，早期診断に優れています。

また，放射性医薬品の半減期もTc-99m製剤を使用しているため6時間と短く，放射線被ばくも少なくなっています。

このように骨シンチグラフィは安全で苦痛を伴わない検査ですので，どうぞご安心ください。

コラム

half-life について（2）

　核医学検査で，半減期についてもっと詳しい説明が必要なときは以下の文章を参考にしてください。

　半減期（half-life）とは，物理学的には放射性核種の量（放射能の強さ）が元の半分になるまでの時間を示す。例えば，核医学検査に最も多く使用されているTc-99mの半減期は約6時間であり，6，12，18，24時間と経過すると放射能の強さは1/2，1/4，1/8，1/16というように指数関数的に減少する。核医学検査を行うために体内に投与されたTc-99mは，実際には尿や便または汗に含まれ生物学的過程で体外に排泄されるので，体内に存在するTc-99mは上記の物理学的な半減期よりも速く減衰することになる。

　Half-life in physics is the time spent for the quantity of a radioactive nuclide (intensity of radioactivity) to become half the original. The half-life of Technetium-99m (Tc-99m), which is most frequently used in nuclear medicine tests, is approximately 6 hours. Furthermore, as time passes for 6, 12, 18 and 24 hours, the intensity of radioactivity exponentially decreases to 1/2, 1/4, 1/8 and 1/16, respectively. Since the Tc-99m administered into the body for conducting a nuclear medicine test is actually discharged by biological process to outside the body carried by urine, excretion or sweat, the Tc-99m existing in the body attenuates faster than the time counted by the physical half-life.

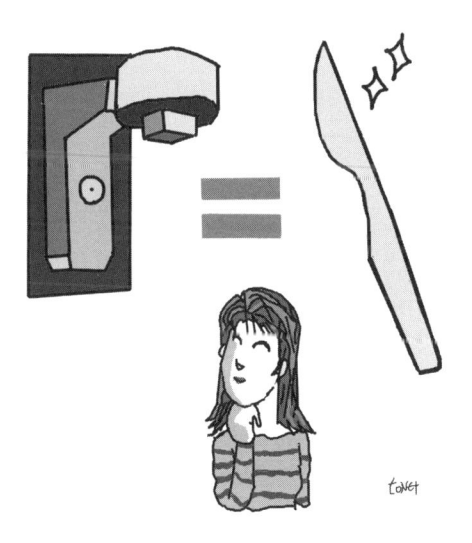

Radiation Therapy
放射線治療

(🅲 2分59秒)

Radiation Therapy

Characters

Pt: Patient   RT: Radiological Technologist

RT Mr. Tanaka.

Pt Yes.

RT Hello! I am Mr. Hirata.

Please enter the Irradiation Room.

RT Now, please take off your clothes from the upper part of your body, and put them into this basket.

Pt Okay.

RT Then, please lie on your back with your head on this side. Please place both your hands over your head.

I think that someone told you, but I will explain it once again. That we will irradiate you every day from Monday to Friday. Because this is your first time today, it takes a little time in order to set the position precisely. It's usually finished in about five minutes.

Pt I see.

RT We will irradiate you in this same posture every day from now on, so please try to remember this position.

Pt Okay.

放射線治療

登場人物

Pt：患者　RT：放射線技師

RT　田中さん。
Pt　はい。
RT　私は平田と言います。
　　なかにどうぞ。

RT　それでは，上半身の服を脱いで，脱いだ服はこちらへ入れておいてください。
Pt　はい。

RT　それでは，こちらを頭に仰向けに寝てください。手は頭の上にあげてください。
　　説明を聞かれていると思いますが，念のためもう一度説明いたします。治療は月曜から金曜まで毎日行います。今日は最初ですから，正確に位置を合わせるために少し時間がかかりますが，普段は5分程度で終わります。

Pt　わかりました。
RT　これから毎日同じ体位で治療しますので，体位を覚えておいてくださいね。
Pt　はい。

Radiation Therapy

RT Some marks will be drawn on the surface of your body. I would like to put some tape over them. It's so that the marks don't make your clothes dirty and also don't disappear. May I put them on?

Pt Yes.

RT Please be careful not to tear them off.

Pt Okay.

RT Because I have to take a radiograph for confirmation. Please do not move.

I have confirmed the radiograph. Please do not move and wait a little while.

Now I will start the irradiation so please don't move.

RT It's finished and now you can relax. Today's treatment is finished.

Pt Can I take a bath?

RT Yes you can. However, please pay particular attention to the marks I drew on your body do not disappear.

Pt Thank you very much.

RT You're welcome.

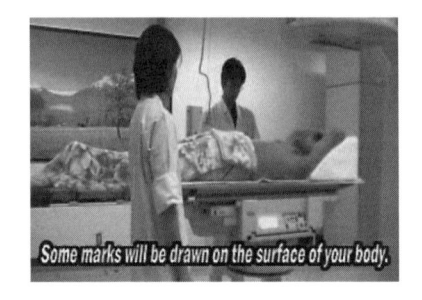

Some marks will be drawn on the surface of your body.

放射線治療

RT　体の表面に印をつけます。体に書いてある印が服についたり消えないようにテープを貼っても良いですか。

Pt　はい。
RT　テープを剥がさないようにしてください。
Pt　はい。
RT　確認のため写真を撮りますので，動かないようにしてください。

　　確認しますので，動かないで少し待っていてください。

　　それでは今から治療をします。動かないようにしてください。

RT　はい，終わりました。楽にしてください。
　　今日はこれで終わりです。お疲れさまでした。
Pt　お風呂は入ってもいいですか。
RT　はい，かまいません。ただし，体につけた印が消えないように注意してください。
Pt　どうもありがとうございました。
RT　どうぞお大事になさってください。

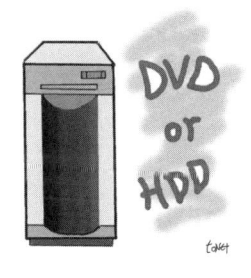

コラム

英語と米語（1）

　英語と米語の違いにとまどいを感じられた経験をお持ちの方も多いと思います。米語は英語の方言のひとつと考えられなくもないですが，移民にもわかりやすい言語とするため，意識的にスペルや発音を変えていったという歴史的背景があります。ただ，時間の流れのなかで発音の変化が進行し，現在の米語は英語に比べて聞き取りにくいと感じているのは私だけでしょうか？

　一般的に，米語のほうがスペルが短くなり，発音に忠実になっています。

	＜英語＞	＜米語＞
色	colour	color
中央	centre	center
宝石	jewellery	jewelry
特殊な	specialised	specialized
劇場	theatre	theater

Influence of Radiation
放射線の影響

(2分31秒)

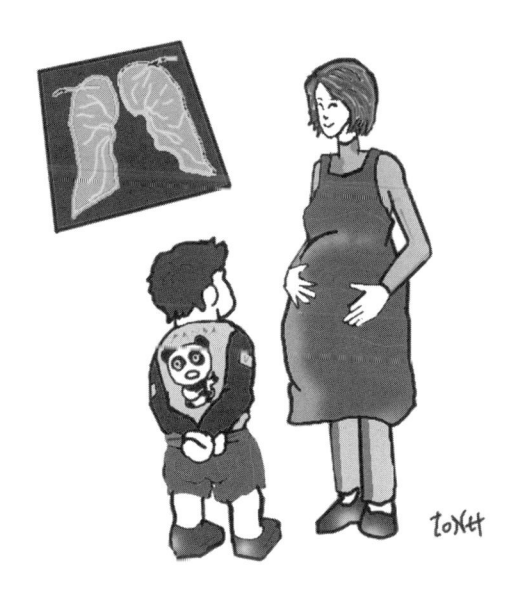

Influence of Radiation

Q Do I really need these X-rays?

A The doctor who ordered them must think that the X-rays are necessary, to be able to diagnose and treat you properly.

Q Are all these X-rays good for me?

A If they can diagnose the problem, the benefits for out weigh the risks of radiation. We do shield the reproductive organs where possible.

Q Do you not shield the eyes, thyroid or head?

A Because they are developed organs, we shield reproductive organs because they have cells that divide and therefore have a small chance of being effected by radiation.

Q You forgot to shield me.

A The X-rays beam is collimated to your chest area only, so there's little to no scatter from the beam.

Q I had a chest X-ray a week ago in the Doctor's office. Do I really need another one?

A The Doctor needs a more up-to-date X-ray that will highlight any new symptoms that you may have and this will aid us in treating you quickly and properly. But I will check with the Doctor if you don't want the X-rays.

放射線の影響

質問 私は，X線検査が必要ですか。

答え X線検査をオーダした医師は，診断および治療をするためにX線検査が必要であると考えています。

質問 これらのX線検査は私にとって害はありませんか。

答え 診断ができれば，放射線を使う利益のほうが害を上回っています。私たちは可能なかぎり生殖臓器を遮へいしています。

質問 眼，甲状腺，頭はシールドしないのですか。

答え それらの組織は発達した臓器です。生殖臓器は分裂しているので放射線による影響を受けやすいため遮へいするのです。

質問 シールドするのを忘れていませんか。

答え X線束は胸部領域のみになるように絞り込んでいます。それで他への被ばくはほとんどありません。

質問 私は1週間前に他の診療所で胸のX線検査を受けました。さらに必要ですか。

答え 医師は現在の最新の症状を見るためにX線写真を求めています。それは新しい徴候を見て早期に正しい治療をするためです。しかし，もしあなたがX線写真撮影を望んでいらっしゃらないなら，医師に相談してもよろしいですよ。

Influence of Radiation

Q Is it safe to have a mammogram every year?

A Generally by age forty, there's probably no risk to the breasts from the screening mammography. Annual screening actually reduces the chance of death due to breast cancer and thus for exceeds any risk from radiation.

Q I am pregnant. Is it safe to have an X-ray?

A Exams such as chest or skull may be conducted safety during pregnancy as long as proper shielding and collimation are used.

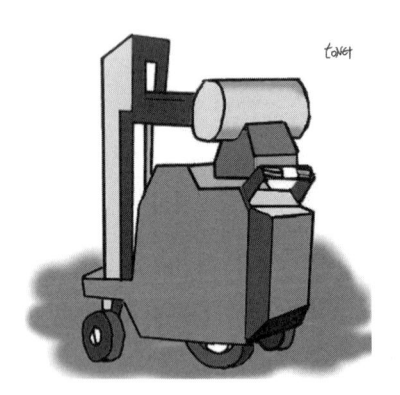

放射線の影響

質問　毎年，乳房撮影を受けても大丈夫ですか。

答え　40歳すぎると，スクリーニング撮影による乳房への害はほとんどありません。毎年のスクリーニングによる乳がん死亡の減少は，むしろ放射線の影響に勝っています。

質問　私は妊娠しています。X線検査は安全ですか。

答え　胸部，頭蓋骨検査は適正な遮へいおよび絞りを用いることにより妊娠期間中でも安全です。

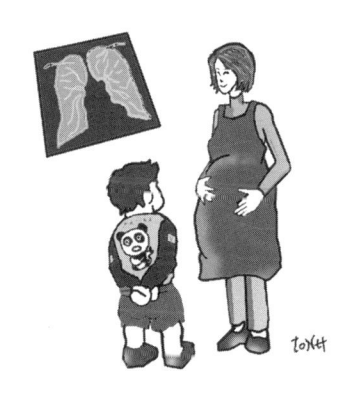

コラム

英語と米語（2）

　スペルや発音が違うだけでなく，英語と米語でまったく異なる単語になるものもあります。なにも難しい単語が違うというわけではなく，普段の生活に密接した単語などがたくさんあります。診療時に使ういくつかの例をあげます。

	＜英語＞	＜米語＞
エレベーター	rift	elevator
菓子類	sweets	candy
一階	grand floor	first floor
二階	first floor	second floor
ズボン	tubetrousers	pants
薬局	chemist's	drugstore
出口	way out	exit

患者を二階に案内するのに，米国人に"first floor"と伝えたら，間違って一階を案内したことになります。注意が必要ですね。また，これらの英国・米国の基本的な違いに加えて，それぞれ地方の出身であれば当然訛りがあるわけで，聞こえ方はさらに異なってくるので要注意！

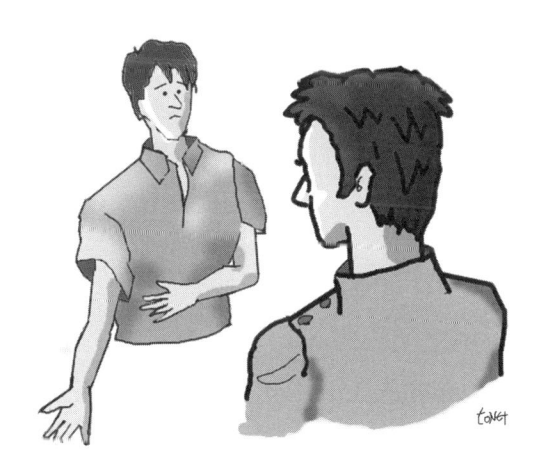

Brief Conversation
簡単な会話

(字幕と音声)

Brief Conversation

Conversation

Hello. I'm Mr. Hall.

Hello. I'm Ms. Mckay.

I'm going to take your chest X-ray. Do you have the piece of paper that the doctor gave you?

(Female) Is there any chance of pregnancy?

(Female) Please take off all your clothes from the waist up, and put on this gown.

(Male) I need you to take your shirt off and any chains or necklaces that you have on.

Okay this way please. / This way.

Step here. / Step on this.

Take in a deep breath and hold your breath.

Relax.

Turn towards me.

Have a seat.

You are all set.

You may go.

Standing (=Upright) or Sitting

Step on this step. / Step here please.

Sit on this chair please.

Face the board and press or put your face against it.

Stand here (over there) and put your back against the board.

簡単な会話

会話例

こんにちは。私はホールと言います。

わたしの名前はマッケイです。

これから胸部写真を撮りますが，先生からの処方箋はありますか。

(女性) 妊娠はしていませんね。

(女性) 上半身裸になり，このガウンを着てください。

(男性) シャツを脱いで，それからネックレスなども外してください。

こちらにどうぞ。

こちらに来てください。

息を吸って止めてください。

楽にしてください。

私のほうを向いてください。

お座りください。

すべて終了です。

お帰りいただいて結構です。

立位または座位

踏み台に立って。

椅子に座って。

板に向かって顔をつけます。

こちら（あちら）に立って背中を板につけてください。

Brief Conversation

Put your chest against the board. Put your hands on your hips.

I'm going to push your elbows forward.

Raise both arms over your head and touch your elbows.

Put your right (left) side face (shoulder, hip) against the board.

Put your back against the board. (Face towards the board.)

Rotate your left (right) side and put your left (right) side against the board.

Lying Down

Lie down on your back please.

Lie down on your stomach.

Turn on your right (left) side.

Roll on your back (stomach), then roll on your left (right) side about 45 degrees.

Body Movement

Bend forward.

Head down.

Bend backwards.

Chin up.

Bring close to your body.

Away from your body.

Point your toes in.

胸を板に押しあてて，両手を腰に添えます。

両肘を前に押しますよ。
両腕をあげ頭の上で肘を抱えるようにします。
顔（肩，腰）の右（左）側を板につけてください。

板に背中をつけます（板のほうに向きます）。
左（右）側を回して左（右）側を板につけてください。

臥位

仰向けになってください。
うつぶせになってください。
右（左）下になってください。
仰向け（うつぶせ）になって，左（右）を下にするように45度回転してください。

身体の動き

ウエストを曲げてください。
頭を下げてください。
後ろに反ってください。
顎を上げてください。
体に近づけてください。
体から遠ざけてください。
つま先を内側に入れます。

Brief Conversation

Point your toes out.

Palms down.

Palms up.

Turn in towards the centre.

Turn out from the centre.

Movement instructions

Please breathe in deeply and hold it.

Take a deep breath, let it out. Hold your breath.

Breathe in, breathe out. Hold your breath.

Relax.

That's fine.

Breathe normally when you're ready.

Holding

Please keep still. / Stay in that position.

Please keep still.

Don't move until I tell you, okay?

Don't move until I give you a sign.

Don't move until I'm finished.

Don't move until everything is completed.

Make yourself comfortable.

Feel free to move.

簡単な会話

つま先を外側に出します。

手の平を伏せます。

手の平を上に向けます。

内側に反ります。

外側に反ります。

動作指示

息を吸って止めます。

息を吸って吐いて，止めます。

息を吸って吐いて，止めます。

楽にしてください。

息をして結構です。

普通に息をしてください。

静止

動かないでください。

そのままでいてください

私が言うまで動かないでください。

私がサインを送るまで動かないでください。

私が撮影を終えるまで動かないでください。

すべてが終了するまで動かないでください。

お楽にどうぞ。

動いて良いですよ。

Brief Conversation

Movement by the technologist

    I have to ～ .

    I am going to～ .

    Allow me to ～ .

    take two pictures of your chest

    push your shoulders against the board

    touch your side

    roll you on your left side

    slide the film behind you

    move you

Movement by the patient.

    Could you ～ .

    Please ～ .

    I would like you to ～ .

    I need you to ～ .

    Hold still.

    Wait until I check this film.

    Turn towards (away from) me.

    Slide towards (away from) me.

    Do this. [*Use Body language or Hand motion*]

    Watch me. [*Show your position*]

    Please don't ～ .

    It hurts when you do that ～ .

技師が行う動作の説明

　　～しなければなりません。
　　～します。
　　～させていただきます。
　　胸の写真を2枚撮ります。
　　肩を板に押しあてます。
　　腰を触ります。
　　左下に回転します。
　　フィルムを後ろに挿入します。
　　体を動かします。

患者さんへの依頼

　　～してもらえますか。
　　～してください。
　　～していただきたいのですが。
　　～してほしいのですが。
　　動かないで。
　　フイルムを確認するまで待って。
　　私に（反対に）向かって回転して。
　　私に寄って来て（離れていって）。
　　こうして。［動作を示す］
　　見て。［体位を示す］
　　～しないでください。
　　～してほしくありません。

Brief Conversation

Move please.

Close your mouth please. / Close your mouth for me.

Take in a deep breath and hold it until I say when please.

Do the best you can okay. / Do what you can okay.

Other

Do your best.

Hold your position.

Wait.

All done.

That's it, all finished.

Have a seat please.

You may go. Whenever you are ready.

You are all set to go.

Take care.

I hope you feel better soon.

動いてください。

口を閉じてください。

息を吸って吐いて止めて。

できるだけお願いします。

その他

頑張って。

じっとして。

待って。

すべて終了です。

完了しました。

お座りください。

お帰りいただいて結構です。

すべて完了です，お帰りください。

お大事に。

お大事に。[明らかな症状，診断のある方に]

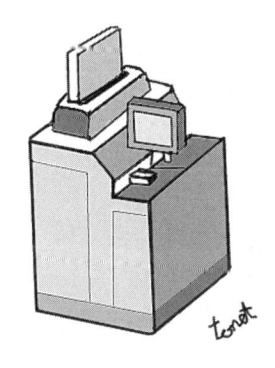

Brief Conversation

Self-introduction　　　　　　　　自己紹介

　　Radiological technologist　　診療放射線技師（RT）
　　Patient　　　　　　　　　　　患者（Pt）
　　Medical Doctor　　　　　　　医師（M）
　　Radiography　　　　　　　　X線撮影
　　Computed Tomography　　　　CT
　　Cardiovascular-Interventional　心血管撮影
　　Magnetic Resonance Imaging　MRI
　　Mammography　　　　　　　　乳房撮影
　　Nuclear Medicine　　　　　　核医学
　　Radiation Therapy　　　　　　放射線治療
　　Sonography　　　　　　　　　超音波

（日本放射線技術学会北海道部会のホームページから一部引用）

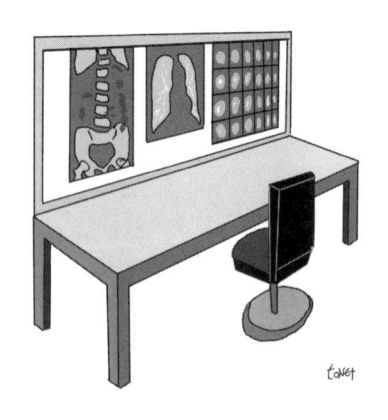

今日から使える放射線診療時の英会話
― CD-ROM 付 ―
ネイティブスピーカー吹き替えによる
外国人への放射線診療時の対応ムービー

価格はカバーに
表示してあります

2003年11月20日　第一版第1刷発行
2020年 2月27日　第一版第5刷発行

監　修　梅崎　典良, 杉山　嘉郎
編　集　社団法人福岡県放射線技師会 ©
　　　　ネイティブスピーカー吹き替えによる
　　　　外国人への放射線診療時の対応ビデオ研究班
発行人　古屋敷　信一
発行所　株式会社 医療科学社
　　　　〒113-0033　東京都文京区本郷 3 - 11 - 9
　　　　TEL 03(3818)9821　FAX 03(3818)9371
　　　　ホームページ　http://www.iryokagaku.co.jp

ISBN978-4-86003-323-1　　　(乱丁・落丁はお取り替えいたします)

本書の複製権・翻訳権・上映権・譲渡権・公衆送信権（送信可能化権を含む）は（株）医療科学社が保有します。

JCOPY <出版者著作権管理機構 委託出版物>

本書の無断複製は著作権法上での例外を除き，禁じられています。複製される場合は，そのつど事前に出版者著作権管理機構（電話 03-5244-5088，FAX 03-5244-5089，e-mail: info@jcopy.or.jp）の許諾を得てください。

付録 CD-ROM『今日から使える放射線診療時の英会話』Ver.2

●ご使用方法
"index.html" ファイルを開いてください。
本編が始まります。次に，左側のフレーム内のボタンをクリックしてそれぞれの動画を再生してください。

●付録 CD-ROM コンテンツに含まれている動画の再生には高い処理能力が要求されます。
必要に応じてハードウェア／OS／ソフトウェアのアップグレード，HTML5 に準拠したブラウザ上でのみ再生できます。
ご利用の PC に音声デバイスが搭載されていないと機能の一部を使用できない可能性があります。

医療科学社のサイトでサンプルがご覧いただけます。※音量注意

（注意）
ブラウザは，Chrome/Firefox/Safari/Edge 最新バージョン，Internet Explorer 11 以上のバージョンを推奨しています。

〈動作環境〉

[Windows]　Windows10/8.1Update/7(SP1)
・Chrome/Firefox/Safari/Edge 最新バージョン，Internet Explorer 11 以上推奨
・CD-ROM ドライブ
・Windows: Windows 7 (SP1), 8.1Update, 10 以降 (Windows のバージョンの確認方法は下記 URL 参照)
　https://support.microsoft.com/help/13443/windows-which-operating-system
・Pentium 4 or newer processor that supports SSE2
・512MB of RAM ／ 2GB of RAM for the 64-bit version
・800×600 ピクセル，32000 色以上を表示可能なモニタ（1024×768 ピクセル以上推奨）

[Macintosh]　macOS 10.9 以降
・Chrome/Firefox/Safari 最新バージョン
・CD-ROM ドライブ
・Mac：Mavericks（10.9）以降 (Mac のバージョンの確認方法は下記 URL 参照)
　https://support.apple.com/HT201260
・Intel x86 processor
・512MB of RAM
・800×600 ピクセル，32000 色以上を表示可能なモニタ（1024×768 ピクセル以上推奨）

※他のブラウザでも動作する場合がありますが，機能の一部を使用できない可能性があります。

株式会社 医療科学社
Copyright©2003-2020 Iryokagaku.co.jp All Rights Reserved.
※記載されている会社名・製品名は各社の商標または登録商標です。